DAPOXETINE FOR MENS GUIDE

Ultimate Guide On How To Use The Dapoxetine Sex Pills For Men Safely and Effectively To Treat Premature Ejaculation

Dr. Grace Thompson

Copyright © 2024 by Grace, Thompson

No part of this publication may be reproduced, distributed, or transmitted in any form or by any means, including photocopying, recording, or other electronic or mechanical methods, without the prior written permission of the publisher, except in the case of brief quotations embodied in critical reviews and certain other noncommercial uses permitted by copyright law.

Table of Contents

- CHAPTER ONE 3
  - Dapoxetine: What Is It? 3
- CHAPTER TWO 4
  - Action Mechanism 4
- CHAPTER THREE 10
  - Dapoxetine for Early Fertilization 10
- CHAPTER FOUR 15
  - Common Side Effects 15
- CHAPTER FIVE 20
  - Interactions Between Drugs 20
- CHAPTER SIX 26
  - When should I use Dapoxetine? .. 26
- CHAPTER SEVEN 29
  - Summary 29
  - THE END 33

CHAPTER ONE

Dapoxetine: What Is It?

Premature ejaculation (PE) in men is mostly treated with dapoxetine, a short-acting selective serotonin reuptake inhibitor (SSRI). It promotes ejaculatory latency by blocking the serotonin transporter, which amplifies serotonin's activity in the postsynaptic cleft. Dapoxetine is rapidly absorbed and removed, making it appropriate for on-demand use rather than daily administration, in contrast to typical SSRIs used for depression. It is sold under a number of brand names, such as Priligy.

CHAPTER TWO

Action Mechanism

The neurotransmitter serotonin, which is important in controlling ejaculation, is modulated by dapoxetine as part of its mode of action. This is a thorough explanation of how it operates:

Dapoxetine functions as a selective serotonin reuptake inhibitor (SSRI), inhibiting the release of serotonin. It inhibits the serotonin transporter (SERT), which is in charge of allowing serotonin (5-HT) to be reabsorbed into presynaptic neurons from the synaptic cleft.

Elevated Serotonin Levels: Dapoxetine raises the amount of

serotonin in the synaptic cleft by preventing its reuptake. The neurotransmission is improved by this increased serotonin level.

Activation of Serotonin Receptors: Postsynaptic serotonin receptors, specifically the 5-HT1A and 5-HT2C receptors, are more stimulated when serotonin levels are higher. The ejaculatory response is modulated by these receptors.

Ejaculation Delay: By activating these serotonin receptors in the brain and spinal cord, the ejaculatory reflex is delayed, which increases the amount of time it takes to ejaculate.

1.3 The way the body takes in

Dapoxetine's absorption, distribution, metabolism, and excretion processes are all part of its pharmacokinetics. Here's a thorough explanation:

Take-up

Quick Absorption: When taken orally, dapoxetine is quickly absorbed.

Peak Plasma Concentration: One to two hours after consumption is when it achieves its peak plasma concentration (C_{max}).

Bioavailability: Dapoxetine has an absolute bioavailability of roughly 42%, which indicates that 42% of the oral dosage that is taken by mouth enters the systemic circulation in an active form.

Distribution

Volume of Distribution: Dapoxetine is widely distributed throughout tissues, as evidenced by its enormous volume of distribution (about 162 liters).

Protein Binding: Approximately 99% of it is bound to plasma proteins, including albumin and α1-acid glycoprotein.

The metabolic process

Liver Metabolism: The cytochrome P450 (CYP) enzymes, especially CYP2D6 and CYP3A4, are involved in several pathways that lead to the extensive hepatic metabolism of dupoxitine.

Both active and inactive metabolites are included in the main metabolites of dapoxetine. Compared to the original medication, these metabolites have lower pharmacological activity.

Exhaustion

Both the renal and fecal systems are used in the excretion of duloxetine and its metabolites. A dose taken orally is eliminated in the urine in about 75% of cases and the feces in the remaining 25%.

Half-Life: Dapoxetine has a comparatively brief elimination half-life of 1.5 to 2 hours. Its therapeutic effects are partly attributed to the extended half-life of its active metabolites.

Onset of Action: It works best when taken one to three hours before planned sexual activity because of its rapid absorption.

Duration of Effect: Dapoxetine's short half-life means that it leaves the body rapidly, reducing the likelihood of long-term negative effects and making it appropriate for usage whenever needed.

CHAPTER THREE

Dapoxetine for Early Fertilization

2.1 Performance

It has been demonstrated that dapoxetine works well in treating premature ejaculation (PE). Studies and clinical trials have shown how effective it is at enhancing a number of elements of sexual function, including:

Increased Intravaginal Ejaculatory Latency Time (IELT): The time to ejaculate is markedly extended by dapoxetine. Research indicates that males who take Dapoxetine have an increase in IELT of 2-3 times higher than those who take a placebo.

more Control over Ejaculation: Men who use Dapoxetine report having more control over their ejaculation.

Increased Sexual Satisfaction: When using Dapoxetine, males and their partners report feeling more satisfied after having sex.

Patient-reported Outcomes: PE-related distress, relationship satisfaction, and general quality of life have all improved, according to surveys and questionnaires.

2.2 Dosage and Management

Initial Dosage: It is advised to take 30 mg of dapoxetine one to three hours prior to planned sexual activity.

Dose Adjustment: The dose may be raised to a maximum of 60 mg, contingent upon tolerability and efficacy. A healthcare professional should be consulted before making this choice.

Using Dapoxetine: It is recommended to take it no more than once per 24 hours.

Administration: Drink a full glass of water after taking the tablet whole. It can be taken with or without food, though meals heavy in fat may cause a little delay in the medication's onset of action.

Considerations: To rule out underlying illnesses and make sure the patient is a good candidate for the medicine, a complete medical history and examination should be performed prior to writing a prescription for Dapoxetine.

2.3 Tolerability and Safety

Typical Side Effects

The most commonly reported adverse effect, which affects a sizable portion of users, is nausea.

Dizziness: Especially after the first few dosages, patients may feel lightheaded or dizzy.

Headache: Usually mild to moderate in strength, but common.

Diarrhea: Reports of digestive issues, including diarrhea, are also made.

Insomnia: A few users may have trouble falling asleep.

CHAPTER FOUR

Common Side Effects

Syncope: A brief loss of consciousness that is frequently associated with orthostatic hypotension—a sharp decrease in blood pressure—occurs.

Mood swings: Although they are uncommon, mood swings, such as depression and suicide ideation, are a possible side effect of SSRIs.

Cardiovascular Events: Patients with cardiovascular issues should use dapoxitine with caution as it may impact blood pressure and heart rate.

Restrictions

Cardiovascular Conditions: People with substantial cardiac difficulties, such as heart failure, irregularities in conduction, or severe ischemic heart disease, should not take dapoxetine.

In patients with moderate to severe hepatic impairment, it is contraindicated.

Concurrent Use with MAOIs: Dapoxetine may interact negatively with other serotonergic medications and monoamine oxidase inhibitors.

Known Hypersensitivity: Dapoxetine should not be used if there has ever been an allergic reaction to it or any of its ingredients.

Tolerance

Gradual Titration: To reduce adverse effects and gauge tolerance, start with a lower dose of 30 mg.

Patient monitoring: It is advised to schedule routine check-ups in order to keep an eye on side effects and modify the dosage as needed.

Education and Counseling: Patients should receive guidance on managing possible side effects as well as information about them.

2.4 Indications (situations in which it shouldn't be applied)

2.4 Restrictions

In some cases, dapoxetine shouldn't be used because of the possibility of severe side effects or ineffectiveness. The main contraindications are as follows:

Cardiovascular Conditions: People with substantial cardiovascular diseases, such as the following, should not take dapoxetine.

Heart failure history

anomalies in conduction, such as atrioventricular block Ischemic heart disease, which includes myocardial infarction and angina unstable blood pressure, either high or low

orthostatic hypotension or syncope

Liver Impairment: Patients with moderate to severe liver impairment (Child-Pugh Classes B and C) should not use dapoxetine.

Concomitant Use with Monoamine Oxidase Inhibitors (MAOIs): Because of the possibility of serotonin syndrome, dapoxytine shouldn't be taken with MAOIs within 14 days of stopping medication.

CHAPTER FIVE

Interactions Between Drugs

Dapoxetine may interact with other drugs, changing their effectiveness or raising the possibility of negative side effects. Some noteworthy medication interactions are as follows:

MAOIs (monoamine oxidase inhibitors): Using Dapoxetine concurrently with MAOIs or within 14 days of stopping MAOIs might cause serotonin syndrome, which manifests as agitation, hallucinations, tremor, hyperthermia, and coma.

Serotonergic Drugs: Due to the possibility of serotonin syndrome, dapoxetine should be used with other serotonergic medications such as SSRIs, SNRIs, triptans, tricyclic antidepressants, and some opioids with caution.

CYP3A4 Inhibitors: Medicines including ketoconazole, ritonavir, and clarithromycin that block the CYP3A4 enzyme may raise the plasma concentrations of Dapoxetine, which may raise the risk of negative side effects.

CYP2D6 Inhibitors: Using powerful CYP2D6 inhibitors concurrently, such as quinidine, fluoxetine, and paroxetine, can raise the exposure to Dapoxetine and raise the possibility of negative side effects.

Alpha-Blockers and hypertension Drugs: Dapoxetine may exacerbate the hypotensive effects of hypertension drugs and alpha-blockers, resulting in syncope and orthostatic hypotension. Combining these drugs should be done with caution.

Alcohol: Because alcohol can worsen central nervous system depression and impair cognitive and motor abilities, it is best to minimize or completely avoid drinking when using Dapoxetine.

Adverse Reactions:

Like any drug, dapoxetine may have adverse effects in certain people. The following are a few typical side effects of Dapoxetine:

One of the most commonly reported side effects of Dapoxetine is nausea. It might happen soon after taking the drug and have a mild to moderate intensity.

Dizziness: Getting up rapidly from a sitting or laying position can cause dizziness or lightheadedness. This adverse impact is frequently temporary and usually becomes better with repeated use.

Headache: Dapoxetine users frequently get headaches. Their intensity is usually mild to moderate, and they could become better with time or symptomatic therapy.

Diarrhea: Dapoxetine side effects include diarrhea in certain people. Typically, this stomach ailment is minor and fleeting.

Insomnia: Some users may experience insomnia, which is the inability to fall or stay asleep. To reduce the likelihood of sleeplessness, it is recommended to take Dapoxetine earlier in the day.

Fatigue: Another potential adverse effect of Dapoxetine is feeling exhausted or worn out. This can happen, especially in the beginning of the treatment, although it usually gets better with continuing use.

Dry Mouth: Some Dapoxetine users have reported experiencing dry mouth. Using sugar-free gum or sweets and drinking plenty of water will help reduce this sensation.

Diminished Libido: One of the negative effects of Dapoxetine may be a decrease in libido, or the desire for sexual activity. Although it usually passes quickly, some users may find this upsetting.

CHAPTER SIX

When should I use Dapoxetine? Usually, dapoxetine is used as needed, right before planned sexual activity. The following are recommendations for when to take Dapoxetine:

When to Take It: You should take dapoxetine one to three hours before having sex. This time frame enables the drug to achieve maximum plasma concentrations and initiate its therapeutic effects when required.

On-Demand Usage: Dapoxetine is meant to be used as needed, in contrast to certain drugs that need to be taken every day. This implies that you should only take it when you plan to have sex.

Flexible arranging: Since dapoxetine does not need to be taken at the same time every day, it provides flexibility in terms of arranging sexual activity. When you and your lover are going to have an intimate moment, you can handle it.

Food Consideration: You can take dapoxetine with or without food. However, big meals should be avoided if at all possible, since they may somewhat delay the commencement of effect.

Individual Response: Depending on a person's metabolism,

tolerance, and particular sexual circumstances, there may be differences in the best time to take Dapoxetine. To determine the optimal moment for you, you may need to experiment a little.

Dosage Adjustment: If you feel that the 30 mg recommended starting dose of dapoxetine is not having the desired effect, you can talk to your doctor about raising the dosage to 60 mg, as long as it is considered safe and suitable for you.

CHAPTER SEVEN

Summary

The following is a synopsis of important Dapoxetine points:

Dapoxetine:

Function: The main indication for dapoxetine, a short-acting selective serotonin reuptake inhibitor (SSRI), is the management of male premature ejaculation (PE).

Mechanism of Action: It delays the ejaculatory reflex by blocking the serotonin transporter, which raises serotonin levels in the synaptic cleft.

Pharmacokinetics: When taken orally, dapoxetine is quickly

absorbed and reaches its peak plasma concentration in one to two hours. It is extensively metabolized by the liver and has a short half-life of elimination (1.5–2 hours).

Effectiveness: Studies have demonstrated a significant rise in intravaginal ejaculatory latency time (IELT), an improvement in ejaculation control, and an increase in sexual pleasure with dapoxetine.

Dosage and Administration: It is advised to take 30 mg of dapoxetine as a starting dose one to three hours prior to planned sexual activity. The efficacy and tolerability of a dosage change to

60 mg may be taken into consideration.

Safety and Tolerability: Nausea, vertigo, headaches, diarrhea, sleeplessness, and exhaustion are typical adverse effects. Syncope, mood swings, and cardiovascular problems are examples of serious adverse effects. People with serious cardiovascular diseases, liver impairment, or medication hypersensitivity should not use dapoxetine.

Contraindications: Dapoxetine shouldn't be taken within 14 days of stopping monoamine oxidase inhibitors (MAOIs) or concurrently with them. Patients with known Dapoxetine allergy and moderate to severe hepatic impairment should not use it.

Drug Interactions: Alpha-blockers, CYP3A4 inhibitors, antihypertensive medications, serotonergic medications, MAOIs, and others may interact with dapoxetine. Limiting alcohol consumption is recommended.

Timing of Administration: Dapoxetine should be taken as needed, ideally one to three hours prior to sexual activity. You can take it with or without food, though meals heavy in fat will slow down how quickly it works.

THE END

www.ingramcontent.com/pod-product-compliance
Lightning Source LLC
Chambersburg PA
CBHW050034230526
45470CB00003B/1265